HEART DISEASE

Published by Smart Apple Media
1980 Lookout Drive
North Mankato, Minnesota 56003

Copyright © 2001 Smart Apple Media.
International copyrights reserved in all countries.
No part of this book may be reproduced in any form without
written permission from the publisher.
Printed in the United States of America.

Photos: page 5—Indexstock: Mauritius; pages 6, 11, 12, 25, 26—
LifeART, Lippincott Williams & Wilkins; page 7—Indexstock:
Scott Shapiro; page 9—Bettmann/CORBIS; pages 12, 13—Index-
stock: Frank Pedrick and BSIP Agency; page 17—Bennett
Dean; Eye Ubiquitous/CORBIS; page 22—Indexstock: BSIP
Agency; page 29—Reuters Newmedia Inc/CORBIS

Design and Production: EvansDay Design

Library of Congress Cataloging-in-Publication Data

Vander Hook, Sue, 1949–
Heart disease / by Sue Vander Hook
p. cm. – (Understanding illness)
Includes index.
Summary: Discusses the heart, how it works, and the diseases
that can attack it, as well as how to prevent them, detect them,
and treat them.
ISBN 1-58340-026-5
1. Heart—Diseases—Juvenile literature. 2. Heart—Juvenile literature. [1. Heart—Diseases. 2. Diseases.] I. Title. II. Series:
Understanding illness (Mankato, Minn.)

RC682.V36   2000
616.1'2—dc21   99-39171

First edition

9 8 7 6 5 4 3 2 1

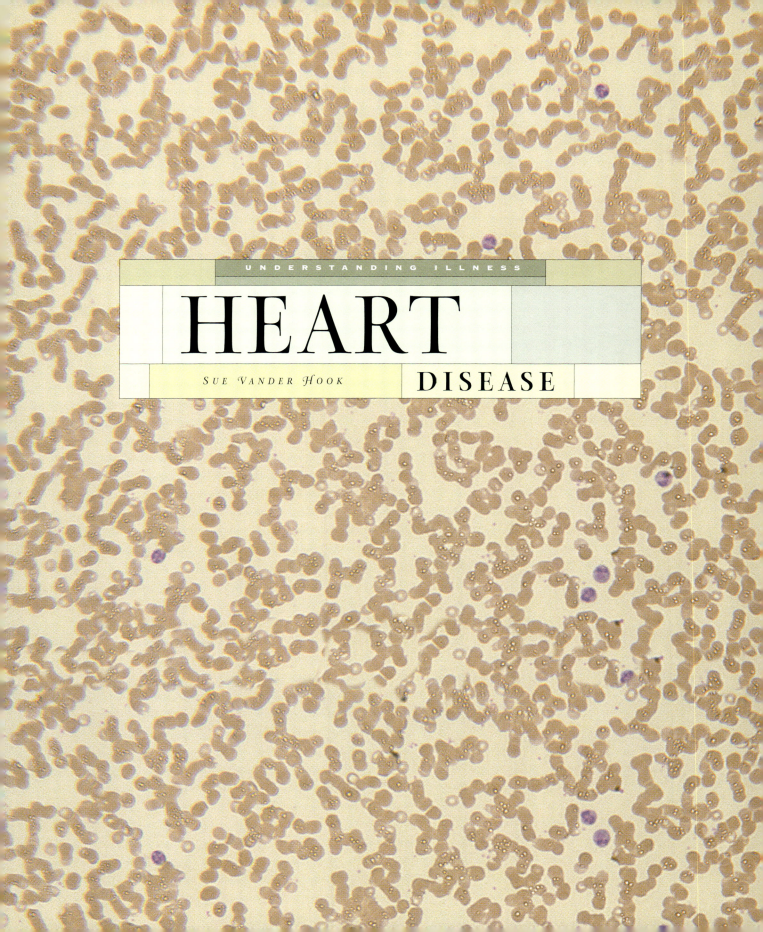

UNDERSTANDING ILLNESS

HEART
DISEASE

Sue Vander Hook

Most PEOPLE TAKE HEARTBEAT FOR GRANTED. YET WITHOUT THE HEART, THE REST OF THE BODY COULD NOT SURVIVE. IN JUST ONE DAY, THE HEART OF A HEALTHY ADULT PUMPS 2,100 GALLONS (7,900 L) OF BLOOD THROUGH THE BODY—SIX QUARTS (5.6 L) EVERY MINUTE—ABOUT HALF A CUP (1.2 DL) EVERY TIME IT BEATS. IF A PERSON'S HEART STOPS BEATING FOR MORE THAN THREE MINUTES, HE OR SHE WILL PROBABLY DIE. HEART ATTACKS, STRIKING EVERY 20 SECONDS IN THE UNITED STATES—AND KILLING EVERY 60 SECONDS—ARE AMERICA'S NUMBER ONE CAUSE OF DEATH. OF THE MANY FORMS OF HEART DISEASE, THE HEART ATTACK IS THE MOST SERIOUS RESULT.

THE SOUND OF THEIR

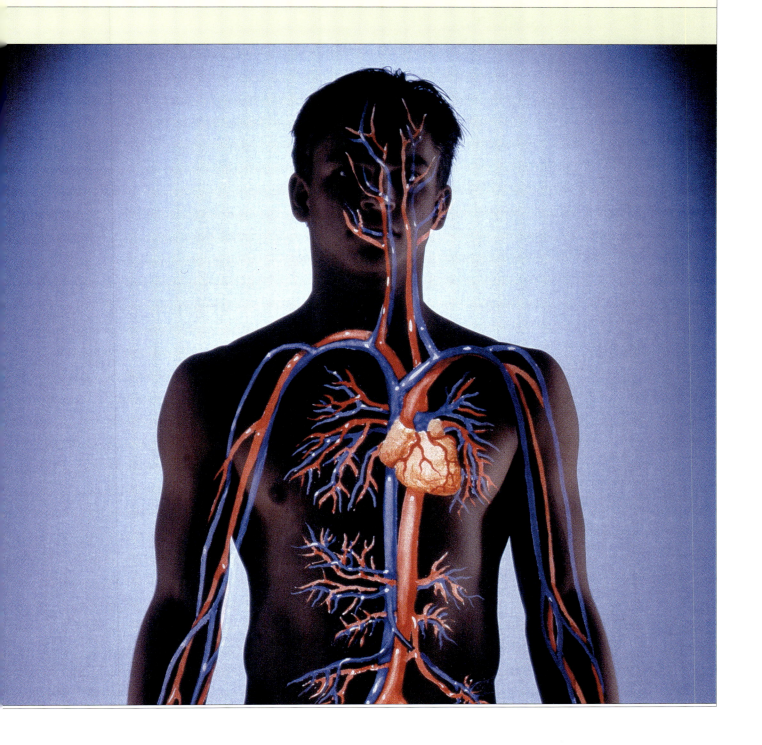

THE PERFECT PUMP

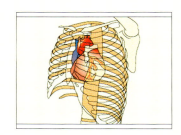

A person's heart is about the size of his or her fist and is positioned at the center of the chest. Connected to this strong muscle is a vast network of **arteries** and **veins**, making up what is known as the cardiovascular system.

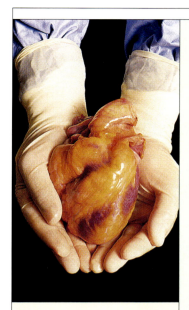

The human heart is not very big, but it has one of the most important jobs in the body.

arteries: blood vessels that carry blood from the heart to all parts of the body

veins: blood vessels that return blood to the heart from the body

atrium: a heart chamber that receives blood flowing to the heart

ventricle: a heart chamber that pumps blood into the arteries

The pumping action of the heart is like the action of a plastic bottle squeezed underwater. When squeezed, or forced to contract, the bottle forces water out. As the bottle is allowed to return to its normal shape, water is drawn back in and the bottle is forced to expand again. Likewise, when the heart pumps blood out, it contracts. As more blood is then drawn in, the heart expands.

The heart is divided into four hollow sections called chambers—an **atrium** on top and a **ventricle** beneath on each side. The right ventricle begins the pumping process by sending blood to the lungs, where it picks up a generous supply of **oxygen**. The oxygen-rich blood then returns to the left atrium. Next, a **valve** in the heart opens up, allowing just the right amount of blood to enter the left ventricle. The **aortic valve** then opens, allowing the left ventricle to push blood to all parts of the body.

WHEN THINGS GO WRONG

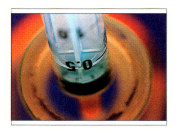

As blood travels throughout the body, it delivers oxygen, **hormones**, and nutrients to every muscle and organ. But sometimes things go wrong. One type of heart problem is **congenital** heart defect. Out of every 1,000 babies born, about eight of them have heart problems that begin before birth. About 25 percent of all

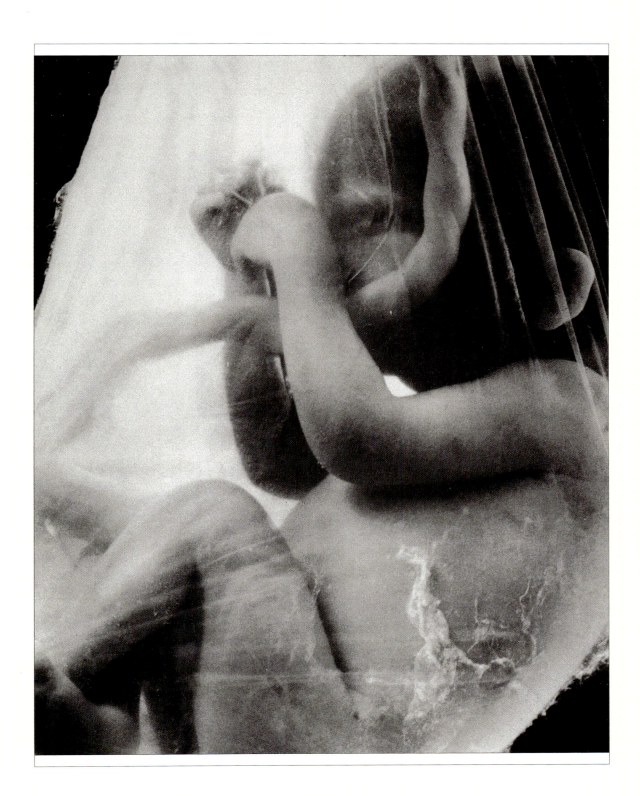

congenital heart conditions are caused by a small hole in the wall between the right and left atriums. If not surgically corrected, this condition—generally known as a "hole in the heart"—can be fatal.

Another heart disease that occurs mainly in adults affects the **coronary** arteries that nourish the heart itself. As the heart is busy pump-

oxygen: a gas that people and animals need to breathe

valve: a passage or opening that allows fluids to go in one direction only

People can suffer from heart problems at any age. Some types of heart defects can be surgically corrected just after birth.

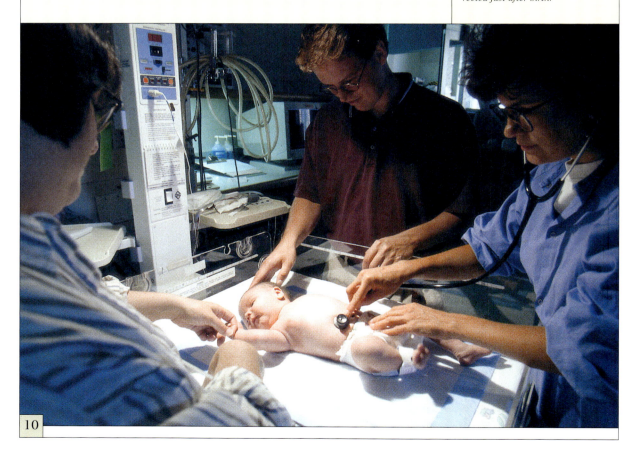

aortic valve: the valve between the left ventricle of the heart and the aorta

hormones: substances that travel through the blood and help to control growth and reproduction

congenital: present at birth

This diagram shows a catheter (a very thin tube) inserted into a blood vessel. Catheters are often used to unclog blocked arteries.

ing oxygen and nutrients throughout the body, it is also bringing nourishment to itself. If the coronary arteries become blocked, the heart cannot get the oxygen and nutrients it needs to function. This problem is called coronary artery disease.

Most often, coronary artery disease is caused by atherosclerosis, commonly called "hardening of the arteries." Over time, as fat and **cholesterol** from food build up along artery walls, blood vessels may become hard in-

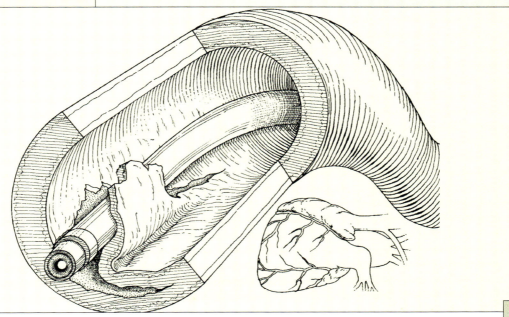

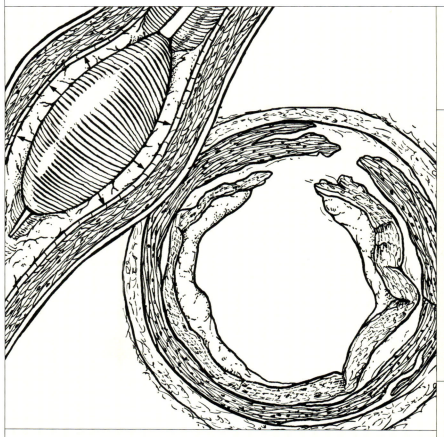

These diagrams show plaque buildup inside a blood vessel (right), and how balloon angioplasty (upper left) can widen the opening in the vessel again.

coronary: relating to the heart

cholesterol: a clear substance found in human and animal tissues; too much of it in the body can clog blood vessels

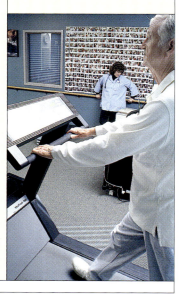

Walking on a treadmill is part of a "stress test" that shows how well blood is flowing to the heart.

stead of soft and flexible. If the hard, shell-like layer of buildup—known as plaque—breaks or cracks, it may block the bloodstream.

Another kind of heart disease affects the rhythm of a person's heart. To maintain a steady beat, the heart relies on natural electrical signals sent out by special cells called myocytes. If

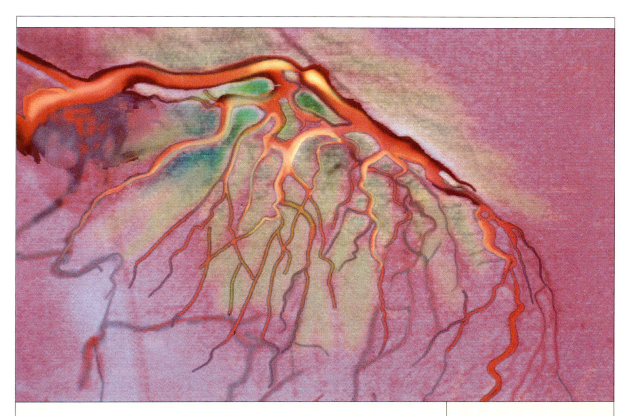

This image shows how fat and cholesterol (visible in yellow) can build up in even the smallest blood vessels, called capillaries.

these electrical signals misfire, the rhythm of the heart may become rapid or unsteady. This condition is called arrhythmia. Health problems known as congestive heart failure prevent the heart from working as well as it should. If left untreated, the result can be a heart attack.

PREVENTION & DETECTION

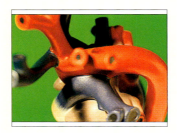

Developing a healthy lifestyle before medical problems occur is called primary prevention. Lowering high cholesterol is one important step in reducing the risk of coronary artery disease. Cholesterol is needed in the body, but too much cholesterol can slowly build up inside blood vessels, slowing the flow of blood or blocking it completely.

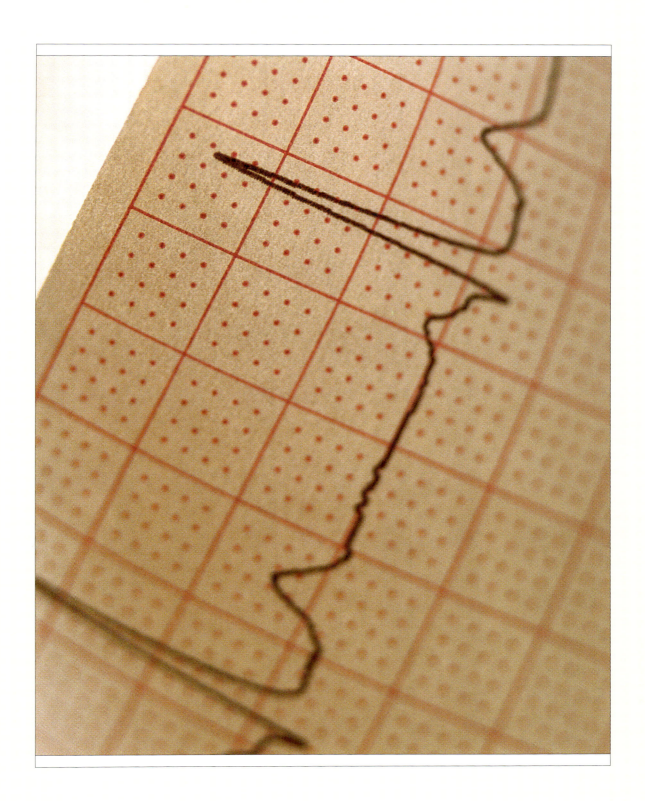

nicotine: a primary ingredient in smoking tobacco

adrenal gland: an organ that releases hormones to give the body energy in times of stress

Smoking is a major factor in making heart disease worse and raising blood pressure.

Lowering blood pressure is another way that people can prevent coronary disease. Blood pressure refers to the force of blood pushing against blood vessel walls. Smoking and excessive worry or stress can make blood pressure rise. **Nicotine** causes the **adrenal gland** to release a hormone that abruptly raises blood pressure, increasing the smoker's heart rate by about 14 beats per minute.

Stress, meanwhile, causes the body to release fatty acids and **glucose** into the bloodstream for extra boosts of energy. These substances gradu-

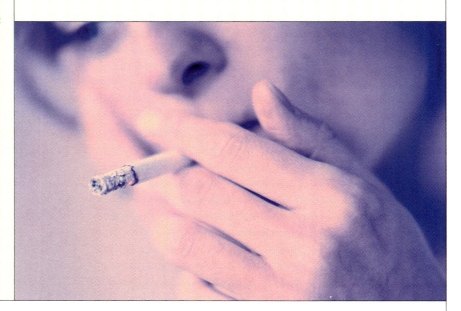

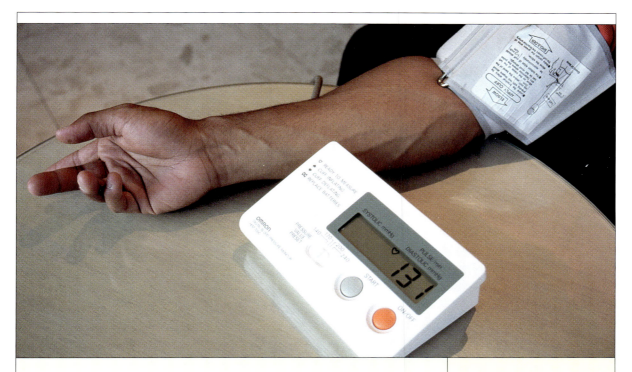

Regular blood pressure checkups are an important part of maintaining a healthy heart.

ally turn into fat and cholesterol, which build up on artery walls. When combined, smoking and stress may increase a person's heart rate by as much as 38 beats a minute.

In addition to healthy living habits, regular medical checkups are also important in preventing heart disease. One basic test, called an electrocardiography (more commonly referred to as an EKG) records electrical activities of the heart.

glucose: a simple sugar that the body uses to feed its cells for energy

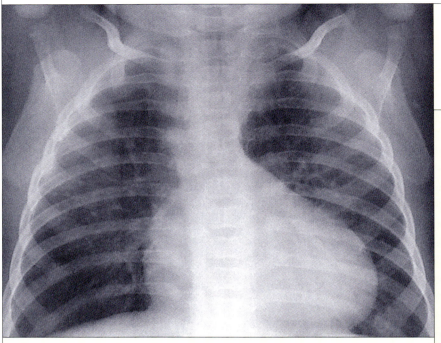

Doctors have long used X rays to look at the heart. This technology forms images that may reveal abnormalities in the heart.

radiation: high energy in the form of radio waves

computed tomography: an X-ray technique that uses a computer to produce images of the inner body

The heart relies on blood to stay healthy. If blood cannot flow easily to and from the heart, the organ may develop diseases.

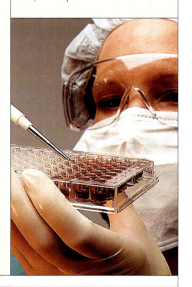

Nuclear scans can create a clearer image of the heart than those produced by X rays or an EKG. To administer this exam, doctors place a tiny source of **radiation** inside the body. As the waves of radiation expand outward, images are created that show the size of the heart chambers and how well the heart is functioning.

Another procedure makes it possible to "look" directly at the heart. Echocardiography reflects ultrasound waves—or sound waves

magnetic resonance imaging (MRI): medical technology that uses magnetic fields and radio waves to create images of the inner body

Computed tomography scans are an important tool in finding heart problems. They provide images of the heart from all angles.

that are too high-pitched to be heard—off the structures inside the body. A computer then receives the echoes of these waves and creates an on-screen image of the heart and the surrounding tissues. Providing even more information are **computed tomography** and **magnetic resonance imaging (MRI)**, procedures that also produce detailed images of the inner workings of the body.

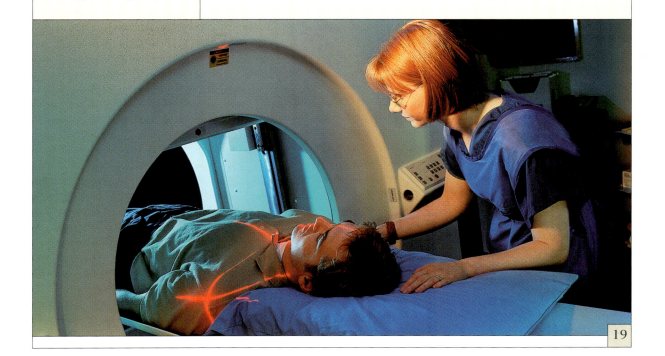

CORRECTING PROBLEMS

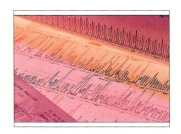

Once a heart problem is identified, a patient and doctor must choose a treatment. Sometimes a **cardiac rehabilitation** program is all that is needed. Other times, medication or surgery is the answer.

In emergencies, the first treatment usually given is **cardiopulmonary resuscitation (CPR)**. If a person's heart has

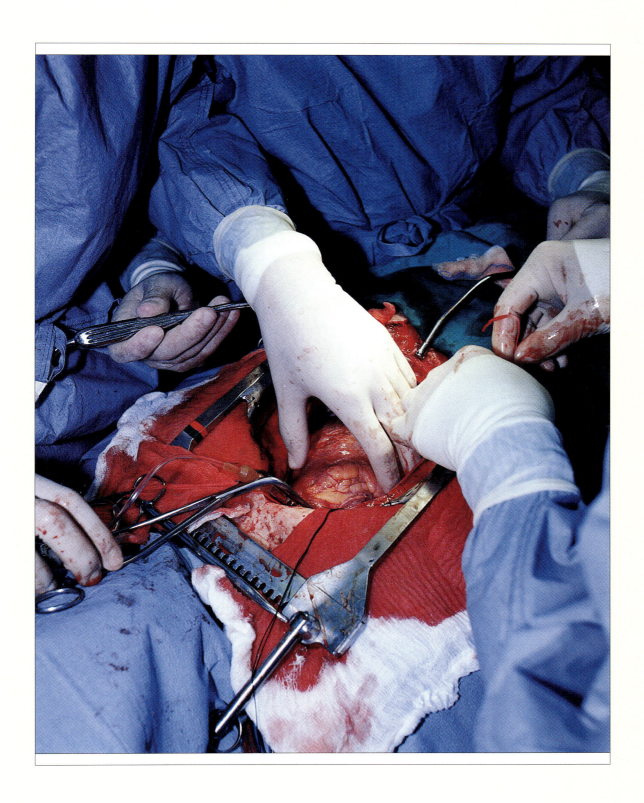

stopped or is beating poorly, emergency medical teams may use a **defibrillator** to shock it back into a steady rhythm. The electric jolt briefly stops all of the heart's cells at once, forcing the heart to get control of its contractions.

Another means of heart rhythm correction is the pacemaker, a tiny electrical device that is surgically implanted in a person's chest. The

cardiac rehabilitation: a program designed to restore people to health after they have had heart problems

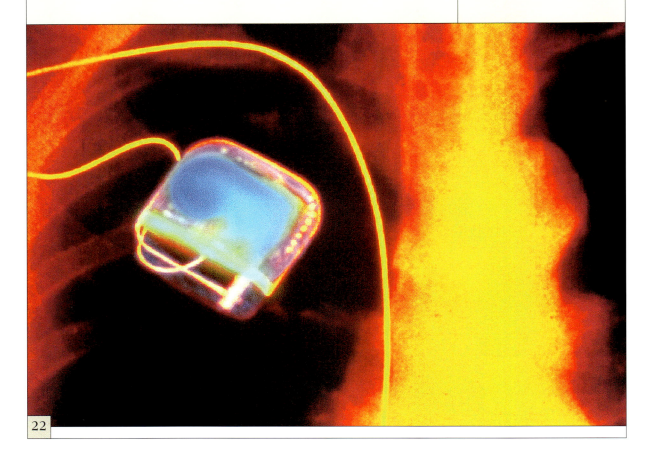

People with especially weak hearts may have a pacemaker. This device emits an electrical impulse to shock the heart back into rhythm when needed.

cardiopulmonary resuscitation (CPR): a procedure to restore breathing in a person whose heart has stopped or is beating poorly

defibrillator: a machine used to send an electrical shock to the heart to control rapid, uneven heartbeats

The defibrillator is a valuable lifesaving tool. Attached to the central unit are paddles that deliver jolts of electricity to the patient's chest.

pacemaker delivers small, steady electrical impulses directly to the heart, helping it maintain a steady beat.

Treatments for blocked blood vessels involve several **catheterization** techniques. A catheter—a long, hollow, flexible tube—is first inserted into a blocked blood vessel. In one method called balloon angioplasty, a tiny balloon at the end of the catheter is positioned at the site of the blockage. It is then inflated to press against the plaque and widen the artery.

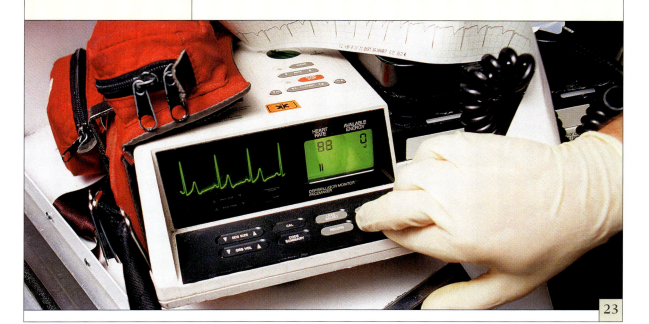

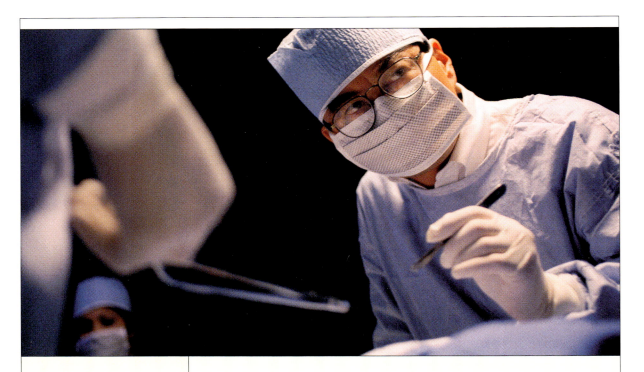

In some cases, heart diseases may require surgery. Although risky, most forms of heart surgery today are performed with great success.

catheterization: a procedure in which a long tube is inserted into the body to open blocked arteries

Surgery often must be used to treat serious heart problems. One of the most common procedures is coronary bypass surgery. Much like a detour around a traffic jam, a coronary bypass goes around part of a coronary artery that has become blocked. The blood vessel used for the bypass is usually taken from the leg or another part of the chest. The surgeon attaches one end of the vessel to the **aorta** and the other to the coronary artery below the blocked area. Blood

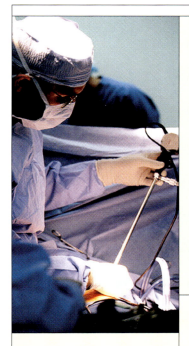

Some people need heart bypass surgery late in life. This procedure strengthens the heart by rerouting its flow of blood.

aorta: the large artery that carries blood from the heart and branches off into many smaller arteries

This diagram shows a heart after bypass surgery. A long blood vessel has been attached to replace vessels that have become blocked.

then uses this new path to once again flow freely to the heart.

In some cases, the heart becomes so weak or damaged that it cannot be fixed, and a heart transplant—provided by someone who has recently died and donated the organ—is the only possible treatment. Because the body

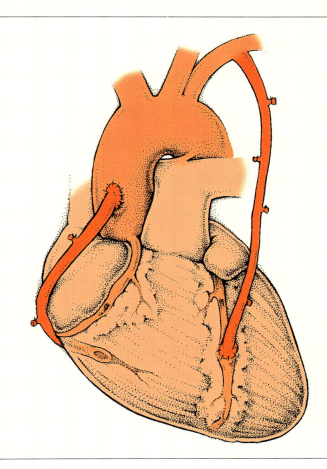

25

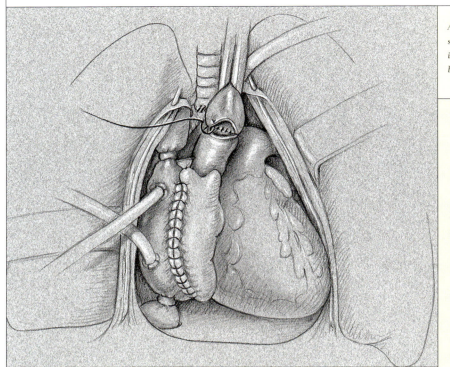

A heart transplant is a complicated surgery. After the new heart is sewn into place, all blood vessels must be reattached.

immune system: parts of the body that resist infection and fight disease

Researchers are constantly searching for new solutions for heart disease.

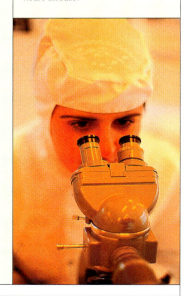

recognizes the transplanted heart as a foreign object, the **immune system** fights against it. The transplant patient must take medication to make his or her body accept the new organ.

Along with other continued heart research, transplant scientists continue searching for ways to use animal cells and organs in human transplants. Every day, scientists, researchers, and doctors continue to find ways to further reduce death and disability from heart disease. But many problems of the heart could be avoided with a few simple changes in the way people live. After all, exercise, a healthy diet, and regular checkups are a small price to pay for a strong and reliable heart.

Regular exercise, such as walking or jogging, is one of the best things people can do to protect the health of their heart.

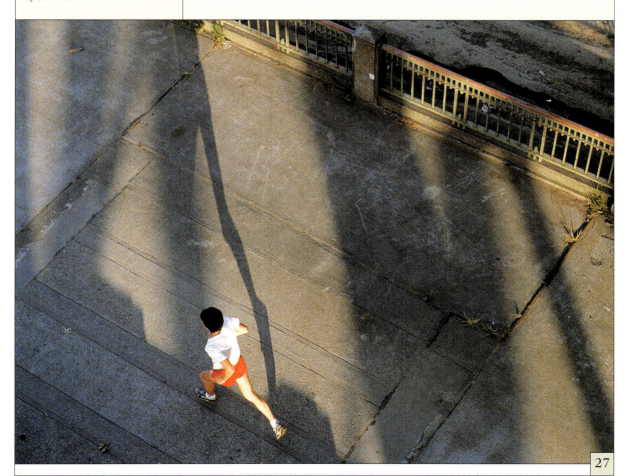

OVERCOMING ILLNESS

Bill Parcells
FORMER PRO FOOTBALL HEAD COACH

Football is known as a physically demanding sport. Although most of the game's injuries happen on the field, football's stressful intensity can affect non-athletes as well. One such person is Bill Parcells, former head coach of the National Football League's (NFL) New York Jets.

Bill, who also formerly coached the New York Giants and New England Patriots, put together an impressive coaching career. Twice he led the Giants to Super Bowl victories. He then took the struggling Patriots to an American Football Conference (AFC) championship and a trip to Super Bowl XXXI. In 1997, Bill led the Jets to one of the biggest single-season improvements in pro football history. In 1986 and 1989, he was named the NFL Coach of the Year. This great success, however, came at a cost to

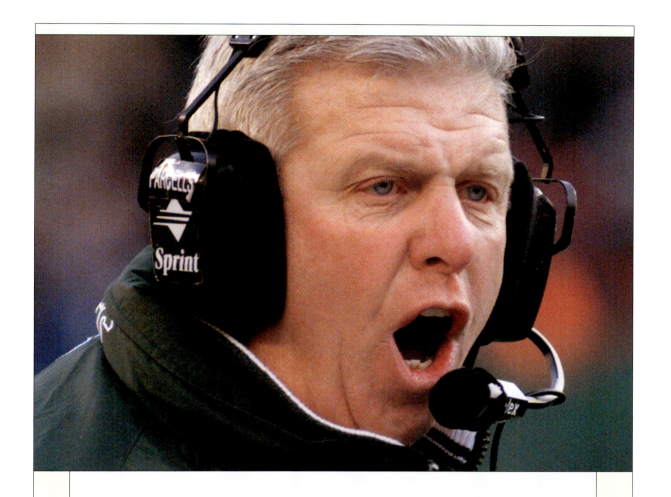

his health. While coaching three pro teams, Bill had four heart procedures.

After having coronary bypass surgery in 1992, Bill left his stressful coaching position for a job as a television sports analyst. After receiving medical clearance from his doctors, he went back to coaching in 1993. In the years that followed, still not free of heart problems, Bill tested his physical condition every day. "I talk to my cardiologist almost every week," he said. "He wants to know how I'm doing at the games."

Bill's hard-driving coaching style won a lot of football games, and a love of competition kept him coming back to the sidelines year after year. Still, he was forced to learn his physical limits. At his doctor's recommendation, Bill declined the opportunity to coach in the 1999 Pro Bowl in Hawaii. Finally, early in the year 2000, Bill decided to end his brilliant coaching career.

The ongoing problems of living with heart disease have not always been easy for Bill. "You can go through periods of depression," he said. "[Coronary bypass surgery] isn't some small operation. You never know how you're doing."

If asked how he is doing, Bill would probably say that he is winning. He has definitely proven himself a winner at the game of football, even as he has continued to do battle with his toughest opponent—heart disease.

ORGANIZATIONS

The American Heart Association
7272 Greenville Avenue
Dallas, TX 75231   www.americanheart.org

Centers for Disease Control and Prevention
Department of Health and Human Services
Hubert H. Humphrey Building
200 Independence Avenue SW
Room 746G
Washington, DC 20201   www.cdc.gov

Children's Heart Society
Box 52088
Garneau Postal Outlet
Edmonton, AB T6G 2T5   www.childrensheart.org

Heart and Stroke Foundation of Canada
222 Queen Street
Suite 1402
Ottawa, ON K1P 5V9   www.hsf.ca

The National Heart, Lung, and Blood Institute
National Institutes of Health
U.S. Department of Health and Human Services
Bethesda, MD 20892   www.nhlbi.nih.gov

The Texas Heart Institute
P.O. Box 20345
Houston, TX 77225   www.tmc.edu/thi/

INDEX

A
adrenal gland 16
aorta 24–25

B
blood pressure 16, 17
blood vessels 11–12, 14, 16, 23

C
cholesterol 11–12, 14
computed tomography 18, 19
coronary arteries 10–12

D
defibrillator 22, 23

E
echocardiography 18
electrocardiography (EKG) 17, 18

G
glucose 16, 17

H
heart problems
  kinds
    arrhythmia 12–13
    atherosclerosis 11–12
    congenital heart defects 8–10
    coronary artery disease 11–12, 14, 16
      causes of 14, 16–17
    heart attack 4, 13
  treatments
    balloon angioplasty 12, 23
    cardiopulmonary resuscitation (CPR) 20, 23
    catheterization 11, 23, 24
    surgery 10, 20, 22–26, 29
      coronary bypass 24–25, 29
      transplant 25, 26
heartbeat 4, 7, 12–13, 16–17, 22–23
hormones 8, 11, 16

I
immune system 26

M
magnetic resonance imaging (MRI) 19
myocytes 12–13

N
nicotine 16
nuclear scans 18

O
oxygen 7, 8, 10

P
pacemakers 22–23
Parcells, Bill 28–30
primary prevention 14, 16–19, 27

S
stress 16